Energize After 50

Energize After 50

Mira Thornfield

CONTENTS

	Book Review	1
	Introduction	2
1	Section 1: The Importance of Nutrition	4
2	Section 2: Energizing Breakfast Options	8
3	Section 3: Power-Packed Lunch Ideas	12
4	Section 4: Nourishing Dinner Recipes	16
5	Section 5: Snacks to Boost Energy Levels	23
6	Section 6: Hydration and Beverages	27
7	Section 7: Superfoods for Vitality	30
8	Section 8: Mindful Eating and Portion Control	34
9	Section 9: Supplements and Vitamins for Energy	38
10	Section 10: Exercise and Energy	42
	Conclusion	46

Copyright © 2025 by Mira Thornfield
All rights reserved. No part of this book may be reproduced in any manner whatsoever without written permission except in the case of brief quotations embodied in critical articles and reviews.
First Printing, 2025

Book Review

Energize After 50: Foods That Fuel Your Life by Mira Thornfield is a treasure trove of wisdom for anyone seeking vitality and better health beyond the age of 50. Packed with actionable advice, the book covers every aspect of wellness, from what to eat and how to eat it, to how to incorporate movement into daily life for sustained energy.

What truly sets this book apart is its approachable tone and practical guidance. Mira Thornfield's expertise shines through as she explains complex nutritional concepts with clarity and warmth. The chapters on superfoods, hydration, and mindful eating are especially enlightening, offering tips that can be immediately implemented. Each section is like a roadmap to a healthier, happier, and more vibrant life.

The inclusion of delicious meal ideas, easy exercises, and guidance on supplements makes this book a must-have resource. Whether you're looking to boost your energy, manage weight, or simply feel your best, *Energize After 50* is an inspiring and empowering read. Highly recommended for readers ready to embrace a healthier and more fulfilling lifestyle!

Introduction

Good nutrition may not have the power to turn back time, but it can significantly enhance your quality of life. By nourishing your body with the right foods, you can unlock a world of benefits: increased energy, better weight management, and improved mobility. Proper nutrition also plays a vital role in reducing the risk of serious diseases, bolstering your immune system, uplifting your mood, supporting cognitive function, and even slowing the natural process of bone loss that comes with age.

Contrary to what you might think, eating well doesn't have to mean rigidly restricting calories or meticulously measuring every portion. Instead, it's about making informed choices that empower you to live your best life. The profound impact of poor nutrition on the body is evident at every stage of life, but its consequences become even more pronounced as you age. Both your own body and measurable health markers—monitored by your primary care physician—can tell a compelling story about the importance of dietary habits.

This book is here to guide you. Our aim is to demystify good nutrition, helping you understand what it truly means, how much your body needs, and where to find the nutrients that fuel a vibrant, active life after 50.

By now, you likely recognize that good nutrition is essential, but have you ever paused to truly understand the intricacies behind it? At its core, nutrition encompasses everything your body derives from the food you eat—a concept as vast and fascinating as it is complex. As you grow older, the significance of what you consume only deepens, influencing everything from your energy levels to your overall health and well-being.

That's why we subtitled this book *Foods That Fuel Your Life*. We're here to explore the incredible potential of proper nutrition and provide actionable insights to help you eat smarter. The undeniable reality is that poor nutrition not only jeopardizes your health but also accelerates the aging process. Together, let's uncover how you can take control of your diet and embrace a healthier, more fulfilling lifestyle beyond 50.

Section 1: The Importance of Nutrition

Aging is a natural physiological process that introduces numerous risk factors, increasing the likelihood of chronic diseases. These risks arise partly due to the decline in the structural and functional integrity of cellular functions and the body's reduced ability to adapt to stress or recover from injuries. Certain substances accelerate cellular aging, with ultra processed foods being a key contributor. These foods, rich in saturated fats, simple carbohydrates, and refined proteins, have been linked to rising rates of obesity and chronic diseases that compromise both the quality and longevity of life. A shift toward protein sources of vegetable origin, tailored to individual needs, is often recommended to counteract these risks.

In contrast, a diet emphasizing fruits and vegetables not only offers low-calorie benefits but is also packed with essential, naturally occurring nutrients that support health. While nutritional needs evolve across the lifespan, older adults face unique challenges. Physical and cognitive declines often impact their diet and nutritional status, making dietary choices increasingly critical. Unfortunately, many seniors opt for highly processed and ultra-processed foods, which are calorie-dense yet nutrient-poor. Research has shown that older adults consume over 14% of their calories from such ultra-processed foods, which frequently include refined ingredients, hydrolyzed proteins, and commercial additives. While convenient, these foods often replace healthier alternatives, as some older adults perceive home cooking as too complex or unnecessary.

Point 1: Nutritional Needs Change with Age

The nutritional requirements of our bodies are not static; they shift continuously throughout life. For instance, during infancy and adolescence, proper nutrition fuels physical growth, strengthens the immune system, and fosters bone development. Similarly, a well-balanced diet rich in vitamins, minerals, and proteins is essential for maintaining overall body function and preventing chronic diseases throughout adulthood. As we approach our senior years, these dietary needs undergo yet another transformation, emphasizing the role of nutrition in maintaining health, energy, and resilience against disease.

For adults over 50, protein intake takes on heightened importance. Adequate protein consumption supports muscle maintenance, enhances strength, and reduces the risk of falls. Protein also exerts powerful anti-inflammatory effects, benefiting overall health. Recent studies suggest that older adults require nearly double the protein intake (as a percentage of total calories) compared to younger individuals. Unfortunately, many seniors either fail to consume enough protein or struggle to absorb it effectively. Research indicates that incorporating 25-30 grams of protein into at least two daily meals can stimulate muscle growth and enhance immune function. Alongside protein, four key nutrients—calcium, vitamin D, vitamin B12, and potassium—become essential for older adults. These can be obtained from delicious and accessible foods like cashew and macadamia nuts, which are nutrient-dense and energy-rich.

Point 2: How Nutrition Affects Energy Levels

Nutrition is a cornerstone of energy production. The body's cells rely on high-quality nutrients to function effectively, and when deprived, they struggle to meet energy demands. This inefficiency contributes to the development of obesity, cardiovascular disease, and other chronic conditions. Personalized nutrition strategies that consider individual lifestyles and preferences can dramatically improve energy levels and overall health.

Eating patterns that prioritize nutrient-dense, balanced meals supply the body with the calories and nutrients needed for physical activities and metabolic processes. While medical concerns can sometimes cause low energy levels, diet is a frequently overlooked factor. Simple dietary adjustments can yield significant energy boosts and support long-term well-being. Choosing the right foods not only enhances physical vitality but also reduces fatigue, helping you feel energized and capable at any stage of life.

Point 3: Key Nutrients for Adults Over 50

As adults age, the risk of macronutrient and micronutrient deficiencies increases due to physiological changes, reduced appetite, and other age-related challenges. Dehydration and malnutrition are common issues in older adults and can lead to serious complications such as hospitalization, diminished quality of life, and even increased mortality rates. Adequate fluid intake, combined with a balanced diet, is vital for maintaining hydration and preventing malnutrition.

Water is fundamental to energy metabolism and plays a crucial role in protein synthesis and nutrient absorption. Micronutrients and vitamins are also indispensable for cellular energy production, supporting every function of the body. However, aging often brings challenges such as diminished taste, difficulty chewing or swallowing, and reduced energy intake, which can compromise dietary habits. These changes, coupled with the effects of malnutrition, necessitate proactive nutritional support to enhance quality of life and prevent disease progression.

Customized dietary interventions, which consider fluctuations in nutritional needs, are essential for addressing the unique challenges faced by adults over 50. Meeting these needs through nutrient-dense foods and thoughtful meal planning supports not only physical health but also cognitive function, emotional well-being, and overall vitality.

Section 2: Energizing Breakfast Options

Starting your day with a nutritious breakfast is the ultimate strategy to keep a few steps ahead. A well-rounded morning meal provides the essential fuel your brain and body need to thrive. While many factors contribute to maintaining brain health, breakfast plays a pivotal role in honing the skills required to navigate life effortlessly. Planning your breakfast the night before ensures you're prepared to make choices that enhance energy management and brainpower. Opting to "eat on the run" undermines the ability to feel alert, happy, and relationally connected to others. Instead, a thoughtfully chosen breakfast can help you take control of your mood and long-term brain health, setting a positive tone for the rest of the day.

"Breakfast like a queen" is a saying worth adopting. Including fresh fruits, 100% whole grains, high-fiber cereals, dairy or fortified alternatives, and lean protein ensures a nourishing start to the day. A poached egg, seasoned with herbs instead of salt, is an excellent choice for savory breakfast lovers. For those who prefer something quicker or sweeter, consider a frozen waffle topped with concentrated fruit spread, paired with plain yogurt mixed with toasted oats and fresh fruit. A protein shake made with yogurt, kefir, or milk, blended with berries, works as a convenient alternative. However, the timeless breakfast champion for energy and brain support remains **hot oatmeal**.

Point 1: High-Fiber Cereals and Whole Grains

Whole grains are nutritional powerhouses that deliver remarkable health benefits, shielding you from heart disease, high cholesterol, hypertension, diabetes, and even gum disease. Studies indicate that incorporating at least four servings of whole grains daily can contribute to a longer, healthier life. One serving equates to options like a slice of whole-grain bread, ½ cup of cooked brown rice or oatmeal, or 1 cup of high-fiber cold cereal. According to the FDA and USDA, at least 50% of your daily grains should come from whole-grain sources.

When choosing cereal, aim for at least 5 grams of fiber per serving. Labels claiming "a good source of fiber" may only deliver 3 grams—so check carefully. Mixing different high-fiber cereals can keep your options fresh while ensuring you get the fiber your body needs. Look for whole-grain breads, tortillas, or pitas made with rye, spelt, millet, barley, or quinoa for variety. Make these a staple in your breakfast routine to fuel your body and brain effectively.

Point 2: Protein-Packed Smoothies and Shakes

Protein shakes and smoothies offer an ideal solution for busy mornings. These nutrient-packed beverages are quick to prepare and versatile, ensuring you can enjoy essential vitamins, minerals, and protein on the go. Opt for minimally processed ingredients like frozen berries, which often boast higher antioxidant content than out-of-season fresh fruits. Organic options reduce exposure to pesticides and genetically modified organisms.

Choose protein powders carefully, avoiding common allergens like soy or dairy if needed. Alternatives like pea, hemp, or rice protein work well for those with sensitivities. Incorporate chia seeds to thicken your drink and add fiber and omega-3s. A squeeze of lemon juice or a handful of blueberries can balance flavors while preventing rancidity in protein shakes. Beyond convenience, these drinks support muscle maintenance, bone health, and overall energy, particularly for older adults.

Point 3: Healthy Fats and Omega-3-Rich Foods

Healthy fats are vital for brain development, mood stabilization, and reducing inflammation. Incorporating these fats into breakfast can enhance cognitive performance and overall well-being. Sources include walnuts, avocado, olive oil, coconut oil, and peanut oil. Omega-3-rich foods like oily fish (e.g., salmon, sardines), flaxseed oil, chia seeds, and pumpkin seeds are especially beneficial, supporting cardiovascular health and long-term brain function.

Adding these healthy fats to your breakfast—whether through a sprinkle of seeds on oatmeal, an avocado spread on whole-grain toast, or fish served with eggs—boosts nutritional value and supports sustained energy.

Point 4: Nutritious Fruits and Vegetables

Plant-based foods are rich in phytonutrients, antioxidants, and polyphenols, which protect your body from disease and promote longevity. For instance, dark chocolate with at least 85% cocoa content, unripe oranges, and various berries are high in beneficial antioxidants. Vegetables such as winter squash, kale, carrots, and spinach not only provide essential vitamins and minerals but also enhance flavor and texture when roasted, sautéed, or blended into smoothies.

Garlic and leeks are members of the allium family with powerful health benefits. Garlic helps combat oxidative stress and supports immunity, while leeks can reduce cholesterol when consumed regularly. Meanwhile, leafy greens like kale and parsley protect eye health by shielding against light damage. Incorporating a colorful variety of fruits and vegetables into your breakfast ensures a range of nutrients to kick-start your day.

Section 3: Power-Packed Lunch Ideas

Lunch is an opportunity to refuel and recharge for the rest of your day, and with a little creativity, it can be a meal that is both nutritious and satisfying. Incorporating a variety of vibrant, wholesome ingredients ensures your midday meal provides the energy and nutrients your body craves.

Spinach Dip with a Twist

Transform traditional spinach dip into a powerhouse snack by mixing ground sunflower and pumpkin seeds for added crunch and nutrients. Pair this with fresh-from-the-oven parmesan thyme pita toast for dipping. It's a quick, flavorful option that combines heart-healthy fats, fiber, and protein.

Leafy Green Salad with Fruit, Nuts, and Seeds

A leafy green salad packed with colorful ingredients like fresh fruit, crunchy nuts, seeds, and quinoa offers a burst of flavor and nutrition. Not only is this a no-fuss lunch option, but the combination of antioxidants and brain-friendly nutrients may also help fend off cognitive decline. Add a light vinaigrette made with healthy oils to tie it all together.

Veggie Burger with a Crunch

For a satisfying, plant-based option, opt for a veggie burger made with grains and vegetables such as lentils, carrots, and quinoa. Toast the patty for a satisfying crunch, and serve it atop spring lettuce, baby spinach, or mesclun mix. When shopping, look for veggie burgers with at least 3 grams of fiber and 13-15 grams of protein for optimal nutritional value.

Easy Egg Salad Wraps

Egg salad is a classic and easy option for lunch. Mix diced celery, unsweetened pickle relish, a touch of mayonnaise, and mustard, then wrap it in a whole-grain tortilla with lettuce and spinach. These wraps can be made in advance and frozen for a quick grab-and-go meal. For meal prep enthusiasts, boiling a batch of eggs ahead of time can make this even more convenient.

Vibrant Salads with Protein Boosts

Salads are a versatile lunch choice, offering plenty of fiber and nutrients from greens, tomatoes, bell peppers, cucumbers, red onions, steamed asparagus, and snap peas. Drizzle with a homemade dressing using healthy oils, and top with omega-3-rich tuna, grilled chicken, lean beef, or roasted tofu for a protein boost.

Forbidden Rice Bowl

Forbidden rice, also known as black rice, is a nutrient-dense alternative to white or brown rice. Create a bowl by layering black rice with vibrant vegetables like beets, Brussels sprouts, and purple cabbage. Add a lean protein source such as beef, bison, tuna, or tofu for a balanced and visually stunning meal.

Point 1: Lean Protein Sources for Sustained Energy

Lean protein is essential for maintaining energy and brain health. Chicken thighs, often overlooked in favor of white meat, provide significant amounts of selenium, a nutrient linked to healthy nervous system function. Just 3.5 ounces of roasted, skinless chicken thighs offer 84% of the Daily Value for selenium.

Other excellent lean protein options include red meats, fish, tofu, and legumes. Protein not only sustains energy longer than carbohydrates but also improves focus and concentration. For those with low energy, incorporating iron-rich foods like lean beef, legumes, spinach, and chickpeas can address deficiencies. Zinc, another mineral found in beef, may help reduce anxiety and enhance mood. Vegetarians can turn to soy products, nuts, and iron-fortified grains for similar benefits.

Point 2: Complex Carbohydrates for Lasting Fuel

Complex carbohydrates provide the slow-releasing energy your body needs to stay fueled throughout the day. Foods like whole grains, fruits with seeds (e.g., strawberries, raspberries, kiwis), and fiber-rich cereals are excellent choices. Avoid simple sugars, which cause energy crashes, and opt for whole fruits and unprocessed ingredients instead.

For example, adding agave nectar or brown rice syrup to baked goods ensures you're using complex sugars for sustained energy. Moderation is key—fruits and grains with natural sugars should be consumed as part of a balanced diet, not as standalone meals.

Point 3: Incorporating Leafy Greens and Vegetables

Vegetables are a vital component of a power-packed lunch. Spaghetti squash, for instance, can be used as a nutritious pasta substitute when paired with a veggie-packed sauce containing mushrooms, onions, red peppers, and carrots. Pureeing vegetables like carrots and pumpkin into soups or casseroles enhances their flavor while boosting fiber content.

Leafy greens like spinach, kale, and Swiss chard can be enjoyed raw in salads or wilted and served alongside roasted vegetables. Avocado, a fantastic source of healthy fat, improves nutrient absorption from greens. For an easy boost in fiber and nutrients, consider making vegetable-based dishes such as quiches, ratatouille, or hummus infused with roasted garlic and onions.

Point 4: Healthy Sandwich and Wrap Options

Sandwiches and wraps offer endless opportunities for customization. Here are a few nutritious ideas:

- **Pita pocket** with hummus, grilled chicken, cucumber, roasted red pepper, and spinach.
- **Turkey wrap** with avocado, tomato, boiled egg slices, and shredded Monterey Jack cheese in a whole-grain wrap.
- **Egg salad sandwich** with shredded carrots and parsley on whole-grain bread.
- **Veggie-packed hoagie** with low-fat mozzarella, sun-dried tomatoes, and leafy greens.
- **Lean turkey burger** on a whole-grain bun, topped with sautéed onions, low-fat cheese, and fresh vegetables.

Whether enjoyed at the table or on the go, these options are balanced, flavorful, and easy to prepare, making them perfect for busy lifestyles.

Section 4: Nourishing Dinner Recipes

Dinnertime is a chance to create meals that are not only satisfying but also nutrient-rich, fueling your body while keeping your taste buds happy. Whether repurposing holiday leftovers or crafting entirely new dishes, dinner provides endless opportunities to embrace balanced, health-conscious eating.

Post-Thanksgiving Sweet Potato Split

Transform leftover sweet potatoes into a creative dish that balances soft and sweet with firm and savory. Begin with mashed sweet potatoes, lightly sweetened with pumpkin pie spice, layered over crispy twice-baked sweet potatoes. Top with your choice of flavorful additions—vegetable curry or roasted root vegetables are excellent options. Pair this dish with a side of red cabbage or leafy greens and something naturally sweet like apple slices, figs, or quince chutney. Include whole-grain bread to round out the meal.

Feeling adventurous? Serve the Sweet Potato Split as a breakfast option, topped with vanilla cashew butter, almond butter, or a dollop of coconut-whipped cream for an indulgent twist. This recipe perfectly illustrates how versatile and satisfying a nutrient-packed dinner can be.

Point 1: Balanced Meals with Lean Protein, Whole Grains, and Vegetables

A nourishing dinner starts with balance. Pair lean protein, such as tofu, chicken, or fish, with whole grains like quinoa, wild rice, or barley. Add vibrant vegetables for fiber, vitamins, and minerals. Whole grains are rich in B vitamins, magnesium, and antioxidants, which are essential for heart health, blood sugar management, and overall well-being.

As we age, maintaining muscle mass becomes a priority, which makes protein a key component of every meal. By incorporating a variety of lean proteins and whole grains, you create a meal that keeps you energized and supports healthy aging.

Point 2: Flavorful Herbs and Spices for Added Taste and Health Benefits

Enhance your meals with herbs and spices that boost both flavor and nutrition. These natural, calorie-free flavorings allow you to reduce your reliance on salt, sugar, and unhealthy fats without compromising taste.

Indian spices like cumin, turmeric, and ginger are known for their powerful anti-inflammatory and antioxidant properties, which can support healthy aging and protect against chronic diseases. Mediterranean herbs such as oregano, rosemary, and thyme not only add depth to your dishes but also promote digestion and boost immunity. Experiment with these ingredients to create aromatic, nutrient-packed meals that are as delightful to eat as they are beneficial to your health.

Point 3: Healthy Cooking Methods and Techniques

The way you prepare your food can greatly impact its nutritional value. Here are a few techniques to preserve flavor and nutrients:

- **Stir-frying**: This quick method locks in moisture and nutrients while maintaining the texture of vegetables. Use minimal oil and cook at high heat for a short time.
- **Steaming**: Ideal for preserving vitamins and minerals, steaming involves cooking vegetables with moisture while avoiding nutrient loss.
- **Boiling**: While this method can reduce certain nutrients, it's useful for fibrous vegetables like cabbage or turnips.
- **Roasting**: A fantastic way to bring out the natural sweetness of root vegetables, roasting at moderate heat preserves flavor and texture.

Choosing the right cooking methods helps you retain the nutritional integrity of your ingredients while keeping meals flavorful and satisfying.

Point 4: One-Pot and Quick Dinner Ideas for Convenience

Busy evenings call for simple, nutritious solutions, and one-pot meals are the perfect answer. These dishes save time, reduce cleanup, and provide balanced nutrition in every bite. Here are some ideas:

- **Hearty Stew**: Combine beef or chicken with seasonal vegetables. Add the veggies in the last 10 minutes of cooking to retain their nutrients and texture.
- **Protein-Packed Chili**: Use lean turkey or chicken with beans, tomatoes, onions, and a side of spinach salad for added greens.
- **Casseroles**: Layer starchy vegetables like squash and sweet potatoes with lean protein and sprouted grains for a filling, gluten-free option.
- **Vegetable Frittata**: A quick mix of eggs, vegetables, and your favorite herbs makes for a simple, satisfying meal.

Get creative with leftovers by repurposing them into new dishes or using them for lunch the next day. Cooking can also become a family activity, promoting communication and instilling healthy eating habits in younger generations.

Dinner is an opportunity to nourish your body while reconnecting with loved ones or simply unwinding after a long day. With a little preparation, it's easy to create meals that are both convenient and healthful, helping you enjoy the best of both worlds.

1. Quinoa and Veggie Stir-Fry
Ingredients:

- 1 cup quinoa
- 2 cups vegetable broth
- 1 tbsp olive oil
- 1 onion, chopped
- 2 garlic cloves, minced
- 1 red bell pepper, sliced
- 1 zucchini, sliced
- 1 cup broccoli florets
- 1 cup snap peas
- 2 tbsp soy sauce
- 1 tbsp sesame oil
- Salt and pepper to taste
- Sesame seeds for garnish

Instructions:

1. Rinse quinoa under cold water and drain.
2. In a pot, bring vegetable broth to a boil. Add quinoa, reduce heat, cover, and simmer for 15 minutes until the liquid is absorbed. Fluff with a fork.

3. In a large skillet, heat olive oil over medium heat. Add onion and garlic, sauté until translucent.
4. Add bell pepper, zucchini, broccoli, and snap peas. Stir-fry for about 5-7 minutes until veggies are tender-crisp.
5. Stir in cooked quinoa, soy sauce, and sesame oil. Mix well.
6. Season with salt and pepper to taste. Garnish with sesame seeds and serve.

2. Baked Salmon with Lemon and Herbs
Ingredients:

- 4 salmon fillets
- 2 lemons, sliced
- 2 tbsp olive oil
- 2 garlic cloves, minced
- 1 tsp dried thyme
- 1 tsp dried rosemary
- Salt and pepper to taste
- Fresh parsley for garnish

Instructions:

1. Preheat oven to 375°F (190°C).
2. Place salmon fillets on a baking sheet lined with parchment paper.
3. Drizzle olive oil over the fillets and sprinkle with minced garlic, thyme, rosemary, salt, and pepper.
4. Lay lemon slices on top of the salmon.
5. Bake for 15-20 minutes, or until the salmon is cooked through and flakes easily with a fork.

6. Garnish with fresh parsley and serve with your favorite side dish.

3. Chickpea and Spinach Curry
Ingredients:

- 1 tbsp olive oil
- 1 onion, chopped
- 2 garlic cloves, minced
- 1 tbsp ginger, minced
- 1 tbsp curry powder
- 1 tsp ground cumin
- 1 tsp ground coriander
- 1 can (14 oz) diced tomatoes
- 1 can (14 oz) coconut milk
- 2 cans (14 oz each) chickpeas, drained and rinsed
- 4 cups fresh spinach
- Salt and pepper to taste
- Fresh cilantro for garnish

Instructions:

1. In a large pot, heat olive oil over medium heat. Add onion, garlic, and ginger, and sauté until fragrant and softened.
2. Stir in curry powder, cumin, and coriander. Cook for 1-2 minutes until spices are aromatic.
3. Add diced tomatoes and coconut milk. Bring to a simmer.
4. Stir in chickpeas and cook for 10 minutes, allowing the flavors to meld.
5. Add fresh spinach and cook until wilted. Season with salt and pepper to taste.

6. Garnish with fresh cilantro and serve with rice or naan bread.

These recipes should provide delicious and wholesome dinners that are sure to satisfy. Enjoy cooking!

Section 5: Snacks to Boost Energy Levels

Boosting your energy after 50 involves not only eating the right foods but also eating smart. The snacks we choose should contain a balanced mix of proteins, carbohydrates, and a small amount of healthy fats to support sustained energy throughout the day. Whether you are sedentary, moderately active (e.g., 30 minutes of walking per day), or highly active (e.g., 60 minutes of vigorous exercise), it's important to adjust serving sizes to suit your individual needs.

Hydration matters, too. Be sure to drink water alongside your snacks and meals to maintain proper hydration—it's a vital part of energy management. And when planning physical activities, allow a couple of hours after eating for digestion, so your body is primed to deliver energy to your muscles and mind.

Quick Snack Ideas

When hunger strikes, ensure you don't run on empty by reaching for one of these quick and smart options:

- An apple or orange paired with a piece of low-fat string cheese.
- Half a peanut butter sandwich made with whole-grain bread.

- A small container of nonfat, fruit-flavored yogurt.
- A small handful of almonds and a slice of whole-grain toast.
- A 6- or 8-ounce bottle of chocolate or flavored nonfat milk (a great post-exercise hydrator due to its protein and carbohydrate content).
- A slice of nonfat ham rolled up with a slice of cheese and a breadstick.
- A microwaved sweet potato topped with cinnamon or a pinch of brown sugar.
- A whole-grain rice cake topped with peanut butter and raisins.
- A handful of whole-grain pretzels paired with string cheese.
- A small sliced banana spread with 2 teaspoons of peanut butter.
- A small bowl of high-fiber cereal with nonfat milk.

Point 1: Nut and Seed Mixes for a Protein and Energy Boost

Mixed nuts and seeds are portable powerhouses of protein and healthy fats. However, not all store-bought varieties meet the standards for a truly health-conscious snack. Look for unsalted and dry-roasted options with minimal added oils. Reclose the container promptly after serving to keep humidity out and maintain freshness.

For a convenient energy boost, keep a small airtight container of mixed nuts and seeds in your bag, car, or desk. Store any extras in the refrigerator or freezer to extend their shelf life. A mix of almonds, sunflower seeds, and pumpkin seeds, for example, provides a satisfying and nutrient-dense snack option.

Point 2: Fresh and Dried Fruit for Natural Sweetness

Fresh and dried fruits are excellent sources of natural sweetness, fiber, and essential nutrients. Here are some ways to incorporate them:

- Add ¼ to ½ cup of unsweetened dried fruit (such as raisins, apricots, or figs) to cooked grains like oatmeal or quinoa for a flavorful twist.
- Create a quick fruit salad with vibrant, colorful options like red apples, green kiwi, purple grapes, and orange segments. Sprinkle with a bit of unsweetened flaked coconut for added texture.
- Serve fresh fruit as a dessert after dinner—simple yet satisfying.
- For a reheated treat, mix leftover cooked grains with dried fruit, cinnamon, and a touch of honey for a warm, dessert-like snack.

Select fruits in season for the best flavor and price. Store fresh fruit at room temperature until ripe, then refrigerate for up to three days to preserve its quality.

Point 3: Greek Yogurt and Cottage Cheese for a Protein-Rich Snack

Greek yogurt and cottage cheese are excellent sources of protein and indispensable amino acids. They support immunity, muscle recovery, and energy stabilization. Stick to plain varieties to avoid added sugars, and enhance their flavor with toppings like:

- Fresh herbs, such as cilantro or mint.
- A sprinkle of hemp seeds or chia seeds.
- Fresh berries or unsweetened dried fruit.

Cottage cheese contains more protein and less sugar than most yogurts, making it a satisfying, low-calorie option. Meanwhile, full-fat Greek yogurt offers satiety and helps your body absorb fat-soluble vitamins, though any variety—low-fat or non-fat—can provide similar benefits. Combine with fruits or crunchy toppings for a nourishing and energizing snack.

Point 4: Energy Bars and Homemade Granola Recipes

Energy bars can be a quick, on-the-go snack, but not all commercial options are created equal. Many store-bought bars contain excessive sugars, artificial ingredients, or low-quality fillers. Making your own granola or energy bars at home allows you to control the ingredients and tailor them to your tastes. Here's how to craft your perfect energy bar:

- Use wholesome ingredients like oats, nuts, seeds, and dried fruit.
- Bind the mixture with natural options like applesauce, mashed banana, or prune puree.
- Incorporate spices such as cinnamon or ginger for added flavor without extra calories.

Homemade energy bars can be stored at room temperature, making them a convenient option for busy afternoons or post-workout recovery. Plus, they are far more satisfying than many mass-produced alternatives, allowing you to enjoy a nutrient-dense snack without compromising on quality.

6

Section 6: Hydration and Beverages

Water is the most vital nutrient your body requires. With the human body made up of approximately 60% water, it plays a crucial role in all major bodily functions. Water enhances energy transportation, lubricates joints, and aids in nutrient absorption. The impact of dehydration can be immediate and uncomfortable, leading to symptoms such as dry mouth, headaches, lightheadedness, and fatigue.

While hydration is essential at every age, your fluid needs actually increase as you grow older. Older adults face a diminished ability to conserve water due to changes in kidney function and delayed thirst signals. This makes it even more important to stay ahead of dehydration. The American College of Sports Medicine suggests older adults aim for 12 cups (96 ounces) of fluid daily, with males requiring up to 18 cups (144 ounces). Tracking your water intake—such as refilling a one-liter water bottle twice a day—can help ensure you meet these hydration goals.

Point 1: Importance of Staying Hydrated for Energy

Water is the simplest and most effective way to keep your body hydrated and energized. Consuming around two liters (or eight half-liter bottles) of fluids per day is the benchmark, though individual needs may vary. Staying hydrated enhances physical performance, focus, and overall well-being. Waiting until you feel thirsty means dehydration has already begun to set in.

Here are some practical hydration strategies:

- Drink fluids consistently throughout the day—don't rely solely on thirst as a signal.
- Stay hydrated before, during, and after exercise, particularly if activities last over an hour.
- Incorporate water-rich foods, such as fresh vegetables and fruits, into your daily diet to boost hydration.

Hydration supports critical bodily systems, from the brain and heart to muscles and bones. Fluids also help regulate body temperature, facilitate waste elimination, and transport essential nutrients and oxygen. With every breath, sweat, and movement, water is lost, making replenishment essential.

Point 2: Water, Herbal Tea, and Infused Water Options

Dehydration can lead to a range of issues, from sluggishness and headaches to impaired kidney function. To counter these effects, aim to include a variety of beverages and hydrating foods in your routine.

Herbal teas and infused waters are excellent alternatives to plain water. For a refreshing twist, try adding slices of fruits like lemon, lime, watermelon, or strawberries to your water. Vegetables such as cucumber and mint also make for flavorful infusions.

If you experience an afternoon energy slump, try:

- A hydrating green smoothie made with leafy greens, fruits, and water. The combination of fiber, fructose, and hydration offers sustained energy and a nutritional boost.

- A salad with a lettuce base—lettuce is over 90% water and provides excellent hydration.

Your body is 50–75% water, meaning dehydration impacts nearly every system, from brain function to digestion. Begin and end your day with a glass of water (ten sips before bed, ten upon waking). This simple routine supports circulation, digestion, and overall vitality.

Point 3: Limiting Sugary and Caffeinated Drinks

While caffeine can have positive effects, excessive consumption—more than five cups of coffee a day—can interfere with calcium absorption, which is critical for maintaining bone health. Tannins in coffee and tea may also reduce iron absorption from plant-based foods like beans and lentils.

Sugary drinks, though tempting, contribute empty calories and increase risks for weight gain, heart disease, and even cancer. Instead, consider:

- Water with a splash of lemon or lime for a hint of flavor.
- Herbal tea or unsweetened beverages as healthier alternatives.

Moderation is key. Limit added sugars to prevent energy spikes and crashes. At 50 and beyond, keeping extra calorie intake under 150 per day can support better overall health.

Hydration is essential for maintaining energy levels and supporting your body's functions as you age. By prioritizing water-rich foods and beverages while limiting less nutritious options, you can ensure that your body stays refreshed, revitalized, and ready to take on the day.

Section 7: Superfoods for Vitality

A vibrant and tranquil life is within reach when you embark on the path of personal nutrition, nourishing your mind, body, and spirit. Good nutrition not only elevates your quality of life but also empowers you to step away from sedentary habits and embrace vitality, peace, and joy as you age gracefully.

Superfoods are nature's powerhouse, packed with nutrients like magnesium, potassium, and antioxidants that offer immense benefits compared to macronutrient-matched carbohydrate foods. With every meal, you have the opportunity to influence how you age and how you feel. By caring for your body and choosing nutrient-rich foods, you'll unlock the secret to graceful aging and sustained energy.

Cooking from scratch with fresh ingredients is ideal, but when time or skills are limited, opt for convenient yet healthful alternatives—minimally processed canned beans or fish, as well as fresh or frozen fruits and vegetables, are excellent options. Let's explore the incredible benefits of superfoods and how to incorporate them into your everyday meals.

Point 1: Benefits of Incorporating Superfoods into Your Diet

A nutrient-poor diet loaded with unhealthy fats and refined carbohydrates can leave you feeling sluggish, irritable, and unmotivated. Over time, poor food choices can take a toll on your energy, mental clarity, and overall well-being. Superfoods, on the other hand, provide the nutrients your body craves to feel energized, vibrant, and alert.

Incorporating superfoods into your diet can:

- Boost energy levels naturally.
- Enhance mental clarity and focus.
- Support healthy aging by fighting inflammation and oxidative stress.
- Reduce the risk of chronic illnesses such as heart disease and certain cancers.

Making superfoods a regular part of your meals ensures your body is equipped to thrive, both mentally and physically.

Point 2: Examples of Superfoods for Energy and Overall Health

Certain foods pack an incredible nutritional punch. Here are some superfoods to include in your daily diet:

- **Dark-colored berries** (e.g., blueberries, açai, red grapes): High in antioxidants and flavonoids, they combat inflammation and provide quick energy.
- **Cruciferous vegetables** (e.g., broccoli, cauliflower): Known for their cancer-fighting properties, they help reduce inflammation and support overall health.
- **Leafy greens** (e.g., spinach, kale, microgreens): Contain compounds that combat oxidative stress, improve digestion, and offer a wealth of vitamins.

- **Sweet potatoes**: Rich in beta-carotene and vitamin C, they boost immunity and promote skin health.
- **Nuts and seeds** (e.g., almonds, pumpkin seeds): Provide healthy fats, protein, and essential minerals like magnesium.
- **Oranges**: Packed with vitamin C and hydration, they add a burst of energy to any meal.

Aim to consume a variety of superfoods every day, mixing vibrant colors and flavors to create meals that delight your palate while nourishing your body. For an extra boost, end your day with a comforting cup of green tea, known for its antioxidants and calming effects.

Point 3: Creative Ways to Include Superfoods in Meals

Incorporating superfoods into your meals doesn't have to be complicated. With a little creativity, you can transform simple dishes into nutrient-rich delights:

- **Breakfast**: Add chia seeds and fresh blueberries to plain yogurt for a naturally sweetened start to your day. Sprinkle unsweetened shredded coconut over oatmeal or baked sweet potatoes for added texture and nutrients.
- **Lunch**: Mix pumpkin seeds into a vegetable and bean salad, or toss quinoa with orange slices, sun-dried tomatoes, and chickpeas for a Mediterranean-inspired dish.
- **Snacks**: Blend freeze-dried strawberries into smoothies or top rice cakes with cheese and nutrient-dense fruit spreads for a satisfying midday pick-me-up.
- **Dinner**: Enhance soups and stews with microgreens or serve a side of roasted cruciferous vegetables, such as broccoli or Brussels sprouts, alongside your main course.

Remember, superfoods can be tailored to fit your family's preferences. Experiment with different combinations to find what works best for your taste buds and lifestyle. Simple additions like raisins in salads or minced tomatoes with oranges can elevate everyday meals into nutrient-packed feasts.

Superfoods are your allies in the journey to vibrant health and graceful aging. By making these nutrient-dense choices a staple in your diet, you'll build a foundation for energy, resilience, and joy every single day.

Section 8: Mindful Eating and Portion Control

Mindless eating is a common trap. Whether it's triggered by TV ads or tempting aromas, eating without awareness often leads to overconsumption of calories and post-meal regret. Research highlights how larger portions encourage overeating, contributing to weight gain over time. The good news? Practicing portion control and embracing nutrient-dense foods can help you enjoy satisfying meals without overindulging.

In today's world of super-sized meals and endless buffet options, portion control can feel like a challenge. But with mindful eating habits and thoughtful choices, you can transform your relationship with food and unlock a path to a healthier, more energized life.

Point 1: Practicing Mindful Eating for Better Digestion and Energy

Mindful eating is a simple yet powerful practice that connects you with your body's hunger and fullness signals, helping you digest food better and sustain energy levels. To cultivate mindfulness around eating:

- **Set the scene**: Sit down in a calm, quiet environment free from distractions like TV or smartphones.

- **Chew thoroughly**: Aim to chew each bite around 20 times to savor the flavor and ease digestion.
- **Recognize your body's cues**: Tune in to feelings of hunger, satiety, and satisfaction. This awareness helps you stop eating when you're full and avoid overeating.

Eating slowly and mindfully can also reduce stress and promote better blood-sugar balance. When you're calm, your parasympathetic nervous system (rest-and-digest mode) takes charge, aiding digestion and nutrient absorption. On the other hand, eating while stressed or rushed activates your sympathetic nervous system (fight-or-flight mode), which can interfere with digestion.

For optimal digestion and energy:

- Eat **smaller, frequent meals** throughout the day to prevent blood-sugar spikes and crashes.
- Choose **whole, unprocessed foods** that nourish your body and keep you feeling full longer.
- Avoid extreme dietary regimens and focus on balance, variety, and seasonal ingredients.

Mindful eating is an intentional practice that nourishes both body and mind. Take your time, enjoy each bite, and notice how it transforms your overall well-being.

Point 2: Tips for Portion Control to Maintain a Healthy Weight

Portion control is a key strategy for maintaining a healthy weight. While it may feel challenging in a world of oversized servings, these practical tips make it easier:

- **Use smaller plates and utensils**: This creates the illusion of a full plate while keeping portion sizes reasonable.
- **Measure your servings**: Familiarize yourself with serving sizes using measuring cups, spoons, or portion control tools.
- **Read nutrition labels**: Check recommended serving sizes and stick to them.
- **Plan your meals**: Prepare meals in advance to avoid overeating or impulsive snacking.
- **Divide portions**: When dining out, split your meal in half and save some for later.

Visual cues can also help with portion control. For example:

- 1 serving of protein (e.g., meat or fish) = the size of your palm.
- 1 serving of grains (e.g., rice or pasta) = the size of a tennis ball.
- 1 serving of vegetables = as much as you can comfortably hold in two hands.

Eating slowly is another effective strategy. Take your time to savor each bite, and pause midway through your meal to assess your hunger level. This approach lets you enjoy your food while giving your brain time to register fullness.

For those over 50, portion control is particularly important to maintain a healthy weight and support bodily functions. By managing serving sizes and balancing nutrients at every meal, you can fuel your body effectively without overindulging.

Point 3: Listening to Hunger and Fullness Cues

Reconnecting with your body's natural hunger and fullness signals is a cornerstone of mindful eating. Start by asking yourself these questions:

- **Before eating**: "Am I truly hungry? Or am I eating out of boredom or habit?"
- **Midway through your meal**: "Am I still hungry? Or am I starting to feel satisfied?"
- **After eating**: "Did I eat just enough to feel nourished?"

Use a hunger scale from 1 to 10, with 1 being very hungry and 10 being uncomfortably full. Aim to start eating when you're at a 3 or 4 and stop when you're around a 6 or 7.

We are born with the ability to recognize hunger and fullness, as babies instinctively know when to eat and when to stop. Over time, external cues—like portion sizes or social settings—can overshadow these internal signals. Relearning to honor your body's natural rhythms takes practice but brings immense benefits, including weight management, improved digestion, and greater satisfaction during meals.

By embracing mindful eating and portion control, you can create a more intentional, joyful relationship with food. These practices not only support healthy digestion and weight management but also empower you to live with greater energy and focus.

Section 9: Supplements and Vitamins for Energy

Maintaining energy levels as you age can be challenging, and supplements and vitamins can play an important role in filling nutritional gaps. Although a balanced diet rich in whole foods is the cornerstone of health, the aging process can reduce the body's ability to absorb or produce essential nutrients. Incorporating targeted supplements into your routine can help support vitality, energy, and overall well-being after 50.

Key Supplements for Energy After 50

- **CoQ10**: Responsible for producing up to 95% of the body's energy, CoQ10 levels decline naturally with age. A high-quality CoQ10 supplement can support cellular energy production, helping you feel more vibrant and active.
- **Omega-3 Fatty Acids**: Found in fatty fish like salmon, sardines, and mackerel, as well as in plant-based sources like flaxseeds, omega-3s are essential for regulating inflammation and maintaining brain and heart health. Maintaining an optimal omega-6/omega-3 ratio is particularly important to combat age-related inflammation. Krill oil is often considered an excellent omega-3 supplement option.

SECTION 9: SUPPLEMENTS AND VITAMINS FOR ENERGY — | 39

- **Probiotics**: A healthy gut plays a vital role in nutrient absorption and overall health. Probiotics can support digestive health and bolster immunity, which becomes increasingly important as you age.
- **Collagen**: The best collagen supplements are derived from fish and provide type I and III collagen, which are essential for the health of skin, hair, nails, muscles, bones, and connective tissues. While collagen lacks the essential amino acid L-tryptophan, supplementing alongside a balanced diet can support energy, joint health, and even mental well-being.
- **Magnesium Glycinate**: This highly absorbable form of magnesium supports numerous bodily functions, including blood sugar regulation, heart rhythm stabilization, and nervous system calming. Magnesium glycinate is particularly beneficial for easing anxiety and improving sleep quality.
- **Vitamin B12**: Vital for energy production and red blood cell formation, B12 absorption tends to decline with age. Sublingual B12 lozenges or injections bypass common absorption issues, providing an effective way to maintain optimal levels.

Point 1: The Role of Supplements in an Energy-Boosting Diet

While whole foods should always form the foundation of your diet, supplements can complement your efforts, especially if age-related changes make it challenging to meet your nutritional needs. For example:

- **Quality fish oil** supplements provide DHA and EPA, two key omega-3 fatty acids that support brain function, heart health, and energy levels.

- Consuming organic fruits and vegetables may offer higher nutrient density compared to conventional produce. However, if your diet lacks sufficient variety, supplements can fill the gaps.

Supplements should never replace a healthy diet but can enhance it by addressing specific deficiencies or optimizing nutrient intake. It's always wise to prioritize a colorful, whole-food-based diet and use supplements as an additional layer of support.

Point 2: Common Vitamins and Minerals for Vitality

- **Iron**: Essential for carrying oxygen to your cells, iron supports energy production throughout the body. Good sources include lean beef, dark greens, fortified grains, and raisins. Pairing iron-rich foods with vitamin C enhances absorption.
- **Vitamin D**: Known as the "wonder nutrient," vitamin D supports bone health, muscle function, immunity, and even cognitive function. Taking a supplement can ensure you meet your daily requirements, particularly if sun exposure is limited.
- **Calcium and Phosphorus**: These minerals work together to maintain bone health, especially important after age 50. A balanced intake is key, as excess calcium can interfere with phosphorus absorption.
- **Magnesium**: Plays a central role in energy production, muscle function, and stress management. Adding magnesium-rich foods like nuts, seeds, and whole grains to your diet can complement supplementation.

Speak with a healthcare professional to determine your specific needs, especially if you're managing conditions like anemia, osteoporosis, or other nutrient-related issues.

Point 3: Consulting a Healthcare Professional for Personalized Recommendations

Personalized nutrition guidance ensures that your supplement regimen aligns with your individual health needs, medications, and lifestyle. A healthcare professional can help you:

- Identify nutrient deficiencies and tailor your supplement plan.
- Address any food sensitivities or absorption issues, such as gluten or lactose intolerance.
- Design a balanced eating plan that prioritizes whole, plant-based foods and moderation.

Qualified experts—such as registered dietitians (R.D.), naturopathic doctors (N.D.), or clinical pharmacists (Pharm.D.)—can provide valuable insights into medical nutrition therapy and help you optimize your nutrient intake. By combining professional advice with intentional dietary choices, you'll stay active, energetic, and injury-resistant.

Incorporating supplements and vitamins into your energy-boosting strategy can help you feel vibrant and capable well into your later years. Combined with a nutritious diet and guidance from healthcare professionals, these tools are essential for maintaining your energy, vitality, and quality of life.

10

Section 10: Exercise and Energy

Exercise is one of the most powerful tools to support an energetic lifestyle as you age. It enhances physical and mental well-being, improves energy-producing mitochondria, and helps regulate blood sugar. While it may seem counterintuitive, expending energy through exercise actually boosts your body's capacity for energy production. Let's explore how staying active can transform your health and vitality.

HIIT (High-Intensity Interval Training)

HIIT involves short bursts of intense effort followed by brief recovery periods, making it an efficient way to improve physical fitness, mental acuity, and energy regulation. Here's how to get started:

1. Warm up for about 10 minutes.
2. Perform intervals of 20–30 seconds of intense effort (e.g., running) followed by 30–60 seconds of recovery (e.g., walking).
3. Begin with 3–4 intervals and gradually progress to 6–8 intervals over a month or two.
4. Alternate intensities (high, medium, low) to avoid monotony and overexertion.

HIIT not only improves glucose delivery to muscles and the brain but also combats insulin resistance and supports mitochondrial health—the key to sustained energy. Always consult your doctor before starting a new exercise program, especially if you're managing chronic conditions.

Point 1: The Relationship Between Physical Activity and Energy Levels

The connection between physical activity and energy is well-documented. Regular exercise not only boosts physical endurance but also enhances perceptions of energy levels. For example:

- A national study on active older adults found that 27% reported above-average energy levels for their age group.
- Resistance training for 26 weeks has been shown to significantly increase feelings of vigor and reduce fatigue.

Physical activity counters the natural decline in energy that often accompanies aging. Even modest efforts, like walking during lunch breaks, can improve energy and reduce sluggishness. The key is consistency—staying active not only strengthens your body but also revitalizes your mind.

Point 2: Pre- and Post-Workout Nutrition Tips

Nutrition plays a vital role in maximizing the benefits of your workout and sustaining energy. Consider these tips:

- **Pre-Workout**: If you eat a nutritious breakfast, you likely have enough energy to power through a morning workout without additional fuel. For longer or high-intensity sessions, a light snack with carbs and protein (e.g., a banana with almond butter) can help.

- **Post-Workout**: Replenish your energy stores with a snack or meal that includes both protein and carbohydrates. This combination supports muscle recovery and glycogen replenishment.
- **Balance**: Avoid energy spikes and crashes by balancing meals with protein, healthy fats, and fiber. This approach promotes steady blood sugar levels and sustained energy throughout the day.

If you find yourself needing larger, more frequent meals or feeling excessively fatigued, consider consulting a registered dietitian to assess your nutritional needs and address any potential sensitivities or imbalances.

Point 3: Incorporating Exercise into Daily Routines for Increased Energy

Finding time for exercise can be challenging, but even small changes to your routine can make a big difference. Here are some tips to incorporate physical activity into your day:

- Start with **15–30 minutes of walking** daily, especially if you're new to exercise. Walking is gentle on the joints and easy to integrate into your schedule.
- Choose activities you enjoy, such as gardening, dancing, or walking your dog. Fun exercises are easier to maintain long-term.
- Use workout tapes or programs designed for your age group to stay motivated and consistent.
- Set a specific time for exercise each day and stick to it, no matter how busy you feel. A committed routine is key to building momentum and improving energy levels.

For those with limited energy or mobility, low-impact exercises like yoga or stretching can still provide substantial benefits. The goal is to move your body regularly, even if it's at a gentle pace, to enhance circulation, strengthen muscles, and invigorate your spirit.

Exercise is not just about staying fit—it's a foundation for energy, vitality, and quality of life. By combining the right activities with proper nutrition and hydration, you'll discover newfound energy that fuels your day-to-day activities and allows you to thrive.

Conclusion

"What should I eat?" is undoubtedly a central theme of this book, but I hope you've also discovered that nutrition is about more than just the "what"—it's about the *how*. Building a delightful, mindful relationship with wholesome, satisfying food allows you to nourish your body while embracing its natural signals and needs. By tuning into your body, you can sidestep the rollercoaster of cravings and mindless eating, achieving balance and vitality without relying on pills or powders.

Become a visionary of nutritional enjoyment. Experience the simple joy of eating in a way that celebrates life, enhances energy, and satisfies both body and spirit. Trust your internal cues over external pressures, and let the wisdom of real, whole food guide you toward a deeply fulfilling way of living. Eating for life is a thrill—one that fuels not just your body but also your excitement for every day beyond 50.

It is my hope that this book has inspired you to rethink your relationship with food—not out of obligation, but out of eagerness to discover how great you can feel. Your body is prepared to reap the rewards of natural, nutrient-dense meals. Your appetite is in harmony with your needs. Your metabolism is working in overdrive, and your taste buds are embracing a fresh perspective.

Now, take the next step. Create a list of vibrant, healthful foods you're excited to enjoy. Dive into new recipes that spark curiosity and pleasure. Just as many readers in focus groups have shared, you'll be amazed at how quickly and effortlessly you can reach your unique nutritional and wellness goals.

This journey isn't about rules or restrictions—it's about empowerment, joy, and living life with vitality. Here's to a future of energy, nourishment, and excitement, one meal at a time.

www.ingramcontent.com/pod-product-compliance
Lightning Source LLC
LaVergne TN
LVHW092100060526
838201LV00047B/1489